HEALTHY WEIGHT
LIVING 95%
WELL IN THE

Size 10 is the new size 4!
Killer workouts, killer cheat days!

DENISE ROMA

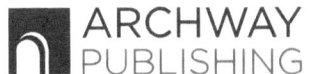

ARCHWAY
PUBLISHING

Archway Publishing books may be ordered through booksellers or by contacting:

Archway Publishing
1663 Liberty Drive
Bloomington, IN 47403
www.archwaypublishing.com
1 (888) 242-5904

Author Photo by John Novi

ISBN: 978-1-4808-4919-8 (sc)
ISBN: 978-1-4808-4920-4 (e)

Library of Congress Control Number: 2017910320

Print information available on the last page.

Archway Publishing rev. date: 07/21/2017

Contents

Get ready for sanity

You may have opened these pages in hopes of finding a way to take off extra pounds. You probably simply want to feel better. Something has to change. Everyone talks about the benefits of eating healthy and exercising; if only both could be done in ways that don't feel like torture! Well, they can. Get ready for sanity around eating and fitness, in ways that feel good.

If you're anything like I was before I lost my weight, you're probably tired of reading books and trying programs that haven't worked for you over the long haul. You're not alone in that. Only 8 percent of people who set out to lose weight do it, and only 2 percent of those who succeed keep the weight off.

Before I found the ways of eating and exercising that brought me to a healthy weight, I was convinced that my body was broken from yo-yo dieting and weight fluctuations. And I was pretty sure that nothing could help.

- ✓ I was tired of dieting only to see the weight come back on.
- ✓ I hated my body and the way I looked in photos.
- ✓ I felt like a slave to food cravings.
- ✓ I saw high numbers on the scale even while going to the gym three times a week.
- ✓ I had rows of diet books on my shelf, but no success losing a significant amount of weight and keeping it off.
- ✓ I was pretty sure that no diet or exercise program could help me.

Yet I still hadn't given up, and neither should you. I learned how to eat, exercise and maintain a healthy weight, and I'm here to show you how. The experience of finally getting it all right led me to the best job I've ever had—helping others treat their bodies with **love** and become the **vibrant, healthy** people they are meant to be. I know if you are reading these words that you haven't given up, and that you *will* get there.

I'm here to help you take on new ways of thinking and acting around food and exercise that involve treating your body with *love* and *respect*. Negative messages about how we don't measure up to media fantasies keep us stuck! The messages that we tell ourselves about not being good or thin enough keep us stuck! We're going to be **rebels** and reject all the messages to hate our own bodies, so that we can actually nourish ourselves and take the right steps moment by moment toward a healthy weight.

I'm 50 pounds lighter now than I was at my heaviest weight, and am now 150 plus pounds of soft thickness and tone. I'm not skinny, and have no desire to be because skinny is not the way I was created.

I'm happy to wear size 10 pants after decades of wearing larger sizes that cut off my circulation. I kept the skinny pants that never fit in those days, by the way-- purchased in the year 2000, and successfully zipped in 2012 (while standing, not in a contorted pose on the bed, trying like mad to get them on, then finally resorting to tying them with string to keep them on!).

Skinny pants aside, my healthy living system is not about being hot, although physical beauty is a natural by-product of the right habits around food and exercise. This is about you saying yes to your health, and no to destructive and false messages about what we should eat and weigh. I'm here with the truth about how to embrace the **original you**, and make it the very best version.

I've often asked myself what sets apart the 8 percent of people who meet weight loss goals. Is it true readiness, and determination, the kind I had when I was ready to leave fat prison behind? What I see in my clients who reach their healthy weight range is a willingness to say yes to themselves, to putting nutritious food instead of garbage food into their mouths and to getting exercise in a few times a week.

After taking 50 pounds of unwanted fat off my frame, and after years of helping my clients do the same, I've learned what works. The best part of my job is watching my clients go from overweight, stressed and fatigued to lighter, energetic and strong. I can't wait to see all of this for you! I promise you that the changes that are about to happen for you will be visible, and transforming.

"And I said to my body, softly 'I want to be your friend'.'
It took a long breath and replied, 'I have been waiting
my whole life for this'." -Nayyirah Waheed

Chapter 1

It's Time to Leave Fat Prison. Forever.

The minute your feet hit the floor in the morning, you are aware of inhabiting the fat prison. You feel it as you take your first steps. You caffeinate to wake up, drink more caffeine throughout the day to stay alert, and eat the junk from the drive-through or the break room because you are not on a diet. Or you are on a diet, so you microwave the low-calorie frozen entree you brought for lunch, which tastes much like cardboard (yet you wish there was more of it). In either situation, you are not eating in a way that is fulfilling or healthy. You're also aware that you haven't been to the gym in months. The result of all of this is that you feel heavy and tired. You hate the way your clothes fit, and at this point, have no hope that they ever will fit, so you rely on the pants with elastic bands—the pants with elastic bands and big, shapeless shirts. The skinny pants stay in your closet out of sheer optimism that a magic thin pill will be invented, hopefully before you get too old to care about clothes.

You tell yourself that a magic thin pill is the only viable option left, because the weight loss programs you've tried didn't work, or they worked for awhile, then the weight came back on. You are sick of the process of starting and quitting diets and gyms. Maybe one day something will click, but for now you'd rather just enjoy your favorite foods and hide whenever someone wants to take photos.

Then the guilt, doubt and desperation resurface. It's time to diet and hit the gym, but you quit after a few weeks because you don't see the results you'd hoped for. Once again, french fries and donuts are your friends, and the scale isn't. You don't know how long you will remain on this cycle, which makes it all feel even crazier. I can describe all of this because I've been there many, many times.

Crazy is behind us now. The habits I'm going to show you are the best of the best ways to eat and exercise I've found after decades of seeing what gets people, including me, to a healthy weight range.

My solutions begin with a shift in your thinking from *self-sabotage* to *self-love*. Self-sabotage happens when you tell yourself that you are destined to be heavy, so another trip through the fast food drive-through doesn't matter, or that you will feel stupid at the gym amidst all the skinny people, so why go?

Self-love directs you to go home and make a satisfying meal that nourishes your body instead of going through the drive-through, and self-love motivates you to go to the gym so that your body can get the movement it needs to be healthy and feel good.

Until you've shifted your perspective to one of self-love, it will be impossible to do the things that lead to a healthy weight *that lasts*.

From here on out, 95 percent of the food you eat should be consumed with the intention of nourishing your body. Eating because "it's time," because others are eating, because there was an ad on TV for food that looked good or to soothe emotional pain are common reasons for eating, but they are not good ones. The other 5 percent will be your wiggle room, for an occasional dessert or other food you've been craving.

We have lives full of social events that revolve around food, and we also use food to meet cravings. It's human to snack for reasons other than hunger, and what you put in your mouth during these times is a big part of what determines your weight.

When you feel the need to snack when you're not hungry, there are foods that you can eat instead of the sugar and fat bombs you may be used to. I'll provide a list of such **go-to snacks** later in this chapter.

When I wanted something salty today, I ate two cups of low calorie popcorn, and some lime fizzly water, which satisfied my craving. This snack tasted good, and was about 1,000 calories less than the movie popcorn and soda I used to order.

Satisfying a craving in a way that doesn't involve putting garbage food (fast food, most chips, candy and overly processed frozen meals) in your body is a sign of self-love. Each choice you make to eat nourishing food instead of garbage food is also one more step toward your lighter, healthier body. You are going to get there taking little steps, taken moment by moment.

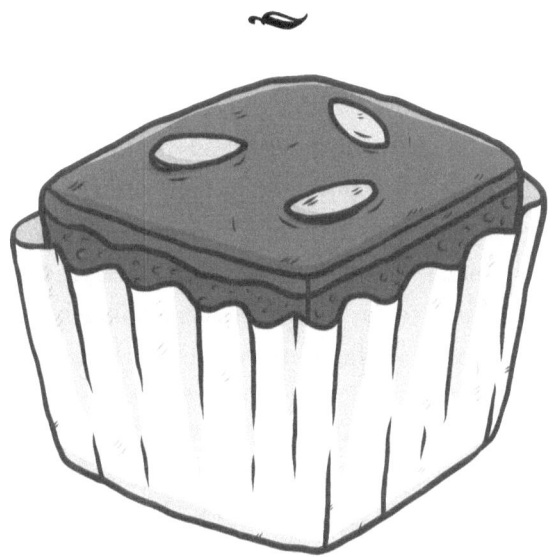

I know all about being stuck in the cycles of diet failure and denial because I've had a lot of experience, enough for a PhD in doing dumb stuff around food and exercise.

During a long phase when I was sixty pounds overweight, I deluded myself into thinking that the following habits were healthy: eating organic desserts almost daily because they probably had less fat, sugar and calories; eating fast food several times a week because it would not really effect my size; and that moving slowly on the elliptical machine was a workout.

My gym buddy during this phase was my friend and co-worker, Tony, whose doctor had told him to lose seventy pounds to prevent heart disease, knee problems and diabetes. We were both thirty-four years old, and knew that it was time to start thinking about our health. On our gym dates, Tony swam laps for an hour, while I got in my lazy elliptical workout.

Tony and I had been reading books about nutrition, and natural remedies. We ate organic foods, and took supplements geared toward weight loss, while sneaking in all our favorite treats.

Tony and I were on our way to the movies one night when he told me that while he'd been swimming three times a week for the past six months, he was not losing weight. In fact, he had recently gone up a few pounds. I could relate, because although I exercised and watched what I ate, I had not lost any weight. When we arrived at the theater, Tony bought an enormous brownie, and immediately swallowed it in a few bites. Since it was 8:30 p.m., I imagined this was the worst time of day for Tony to eat a big brownie. Wasn't he canceling out all the effort he'd made earlier in the day by taking supplements, and going to the gym?

My heart sank as it occurred to me that my eating habits were just as counter-intuitive to my own goals. My bad habits had been going on for years, maybe decades, but I had been unwilling to admit it to myself. I'd had my own version of the night of the big brownie many times.

I was not behaving in ways that resulted in a healthy weight at all. For a 5'5", small-boned person, 195 wasn't a good number for me to see on the scale.

Even though it was tough to admit that my own choices were keeping my weight much too high, until I owned that my size was the result of my own behavior, nothing could change—not my weight, not feeling like crap and not the maddening cycles of dieting, exercising and getting nowhere.

Carrying more than a few extra pounds hurt for me, and it hurts for you. The heart wears out pumping blood to miles of additional arteries, joints ache from doing the work of carrying extra weight, and self-esteem suffers big time.

The emotions heavy people experience are heavy, too; shame, frustration, hopelessness and loneliness are common. For those who are significantly overweight, there is also isolation and immobility. That's why I call it fat prison.

You leave fat prison when you start eating real food, and when you give your body the movement it needs. I promise you that once you start truly caring for your body through nutritious eating and movement that you will feel better. Living well is a lifelong process, and while reaching your goal weight can be part of what happens along the way, it's not an end in itself.

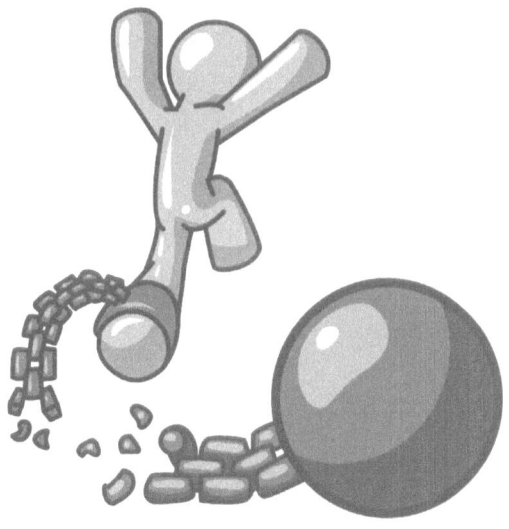

My client, and one of my very favorite people, Sheila, came to me at 219 pounds and a size 20. She had weighed 120 as a college senior, so she was surprised when the weight crept on during thirty years of running her own design business. Sheila was also somewhat lost as far as how to work out at the gym, the same way that I was.

I'm happy to tell you that Sheila has lost forty pounds. She ran her first 5K a couple of years ago; she jogs 2-3 miles twice a week, and gets in yoga twice weekly between workouts with me. Sheila fit into a size 12 recently, and this was extremely exciting for both of us.

What made the difference for Sheila was learning how to exercise efficiently, and how to prepare fresh, delicious meals off the grocery list I'll provide later in this chapter. She made sure these foods were in her environments, and that garbage foods were not. Sheila stopped eating bread with every meal, and paid attention to sugar grams and portion sizes. She added fresh vegetables, fruit and lean protein sources to her meals and made wine a twice-weekly instead of nightly treat.

Sheila and I have agreed that her ideal weight for this phase of her life is around 180. If Sheila wanted to fit into her college jeans, she would have to give up the celebrating that is part of her social and work life, which she enjoys so much. At 180, which Sheila carries well on her 5'9, large-boned frame, she can wear her size 12 pants, jog, do yoga and have energy for life. She doesn't have to shoot for her college weight right now, and she's lot healthier than she was at 219 and not eating well or exercising.

This doesn't mean that I believe being significantly overweight is a good thing. What I want -- for myself, for my clients and you -- is a weight where you feel lighter and healthier than you may have ever felt before.

My own healthy weight is somewhere between 145-155. If I were to shoot for 135 and maintain that weight, I'd have to do without many of the treats I enjoy. I love to have a weekly cheat day where I get to eat a couple things, or three, that I've been craving all week. It's divine to split an order of pasta, and have a glass of wine or dessert occasionally. A small piece of my mom's famous secret recipe cheese-cake is mandatory!

I want to help you take on thoughts and behaviors around eating that are just as realistic. You need room to enjoy what you like in more moderate amounts, while reaching your healthy weight range, and staying there.

I want you feeling better structurally, too. Yes, I want your knees and ankles to stop twinging when you walk or climb stairs, and I also want your spirit feeling better, liberated from the cycles of failure of earlier diet and exercise attempts.

The first step in this liberation is getting your refrigerator and shelves stocked with the right foods. There are great benefits other than weight loss that come from eating nourishing real food, avoiding unhealthy garbage food and from getting consistent exercise. You will begin to notice other positive changes:

- quality of sleep
- better overall mood
- more energy
- healthier hair and skin

Losing weight in a way that lasts takes time, and you should know that other good things will happen very soon!

Unhealthy foods are available to us everywhere. Be ready for the enemy that is the standard American diet: junk foods, fast foods and "regular" food that makes us gain unwanted pounds.

These foods include: muffins that are so high in sugar and fat that you may as well have cake for breakfast; sodas, smoothies and juices that contain 30-70 grams of sugar per serving; and weight reduction frozen dinners or snacks that don't satisfy hunger, and lead to cravings for more sugar/carbs.

First, let's kick the garbage out of your house, and replace it with nourishing food that will fill you up. We are going to get you off the sugar/carb munchies cycle, so that sweets are an occasional treat, instead of a trigger that leave you hungry and craving more.

Here are some examples of what to clear out of your cupboards: candy, any snack or sports bar that has more than 17 grams of sugar, potato chips, muffins, cakes and soups that have more than 500 mg of sodium per serving.

Now go to the fridge/freezer and get rid of frozen entrees or pizzas, ice-cream and anything else that common sense would dictate is not compatible with weight loss. Frozen treats made by weight reduction companies are okay if you're able to enjoy them in moderation, and they don't trigger you to eat more than one.

Next, go to any other place you keep snacks, like the glove compartment or snack drawer at work. Take a bag, and put all of the unhealthy foods into it. Donate it, or throw it away.

Garbage food interferes with your weight loss goals, because your body can't digest overly-processed chemical-laden food well. It hangs in your gut for days, because is not really meant for human consumption. It sounds gross because it is.

Foods to Get Out of the House

What:	Why:
Energy drinks	Caffeine, sugar, chemicals.
Regular and Diet soda	Chemical sludge loaded with sugar and caffeine.
Juices	Almost as much sugar per serving as soda.
Candy bars, chips, donuts	Nutritionally void; sugar triggers.

Now for your next step out of fat prison-- getting healthy foods into your environments by loading up on these foods:

Your Grocery List

Dark, leafy greens like spinach or kale for salads

Avocados

Tomatoes, peppers, onions and any other vegetable you like

Hummus to dip vegetables in

Fruit

Lean meats -- fish, chicken, pork, beef and chicken

Eggs

Turkey bacon or sausage

Chicken or turkey sausage/hotdogs

Organic lunch meat low in nitrates, chemicals and sodium

Whole grain bread

Whole grain English muffins

Olive oil and vinegar, or organic salad dressing

Spreadable butter (use in moderation)

Cheese (use in moderation)

Olives

Almonds, walnuts or whatever nut you like (use in moderation)

Greek yogurt

Dark chocolate (in single servings preferably)

Coffee or tea if you drink it

Spray can whipped cream (15 calories per serving)

Slow-cooked oatmeal

Sweet potatoes (lower in sugar than white or red potatoes)

A thin crust organic frozen pizza (Kashi and Amy's make good ones) to have on stock as a special treat. You want to dig into this instead of dialing for pizza

Natural, low-calorie popcorn (eat in moderation)
Regular or carbonated "fizzly" water

Once you have the nutritious foods on the list, go back to your environments with them. Stock the fridge at work with snacks like cheese sticks, fresh fruit, celery, peppers and little tomatoes. Put a baggie filled with almonds in the glove compartment. With the right foods on hand, you'll never have to get too hungry, and will be armed to fight cravings.

When you get too hungry, your primal brain demands sugar, salt and fat. This is what the fast food places offer in abundance, because many people go there when they are hungry and busy.

If you follow my shopping and stocking plan, you will have a healthy snack readily available to stay out of the line of hungry, stressed-out people who keep the fast food industry in business, and who are also in line for obesity-related illnesses like heart disease and diabetes.

A common a-ha moment my clients have as the fat comes off is that real food tastes so much better than garbage food. Their routine fast food chicken sandwich with fries suddenly pales in comparison to a chicken breast baked or grilled at home on half a whole grain bun with a slice of avocado, maybe a little bit of mayo and homemade sweet potato fries.

The first option is full of salt, sugar, chemicals and drag-me-down white bread; it may have been sitting under a lamp for a while. The second option is fresh, tastes delicious, fills you and doesn't leave you slipping off your goals.

If you protest that you don't have time to prepare food and can only eat on the go because of long work hours or other responsibilities, I'm going to set you straight right here. This is your health we're talking about, and it's incredibly important that you take time to prepare your food. The old thinking, that you don't have time, must go out the window with the garbage food you threw out.

One way of treating your body well is taking the time to prepare food. You deserve it! Of course, it's easier to head through the drive-through after a long day, and I'm not telling you that this won't happen on occasion. You are not going to let those slip-ups deter you, and you're going to reach a point where you will prefer the way real food tastes.

As you prepare your food, and as you eat it throughout the day, remind yourself that your health is most important, and that you are will put nourishing, real food into your body as an act of self-love.

You will notice that others carry fast food bags, sodas and candy bars. After a while, you will feel sorry that they don't have the information you do about eating real food instead of garbage food. You will notice that they have a lot less energy, and often complain about being tired.

We've talked about what is in your environment as far as food and drinks go, but equally important is *who's* in your environment?

Negative people discourage you. No matter how healthy your diet and exercise rituals, if there are negative people who discourage you, and who do not support your healthy habits, then it will be difficult for a lasting transformation in your fitness and weight to take place. Negative people sabotage others by invalidating their positive behavior around food and exercise, or by giving non-verbal messages that they disapprove.

The people to consider reducing time spent with are those who tempt you to eat your trigger foods, who complain about the changes you're making or give you disapproving messages when you don't make unhealthy choices alongside them.

One of my clients, Julie, found that she had to reconsider whether she wanted to keep spending time with her friend, Cat, as Julie began changing her nutrition and started exercising. Julie had struggled with losing extra pounds since her teen years. Her friend from a past workplace, Cat, had the same frame and carried extra pounds, too. These gals had bonded eight years earlier when they met as admins for the same department.

Julie and Cat had been what Cat called the "large and in charge ladies" of their organization. However, Julie had never liked being heavy, and had tried many diets. She had even invited Cat to join her on her weight loss endeavors at one point. Cat turned her down, saying that diets didn't work for her.

Julie lost ten pounds in three months after creating new rituals with me around positive nutrition and exercise. Then it was time to meet Cat for lunch again. Because Julie was doing strength training with me, it looked like she had lost more like twenty pounds, because a ten-pound fat loss always looks like about twenty pounds lost since fat is light, and takes up so much space.

Julie texted me on her way to the restaurant where she was to meet Cat, and asked what she could possibly order at the restaurant. I looked at the menu online, and helped Julie settle on a grilled chicken salad with avocado, fresh fruit instead of french fries, and water with a wedge of lime. Since Cat and Julie always ordered dessert, Julie agreed that she would ask her friend if they could share one.

When Julie arrived at the restaurant, Cat was waiting for her at a booth. They had not seen each other since Julie had lost weight, and Cat stared as Julie took off her coat.

"Whoa, look at you!" Cat said. "Don't tell me you're starving yourself again."

Julie shared her excitement, that she was seeing a fitness coach, and had lost ten pounds.

As Julie and Cat ate their very different lunches, Cat kidded Julie about drinking water instead of soda, and said that Julie was stuck up when Julie wouldn't share onion rings. Julie suggested they share a dessert, so as not to break tradition. Julie had thought this would make Cat happy, but her friend rolled her eyes.

"Whenever you go on a diet, this always happens," Cat said. "Don't worry. I'll be there when you fall off the wagon. Then we can go out for the kitchen sink pizza."

"This isn't just another diet," Julie said, mustering reserves of patience. "I promise I won't try to make you do anything. I just ask that you don't make fun of me while I make some new choices."

Julie ended up keeping Cat on her Christmas card list, but made excuses when Cat asked her to lunch again. She didn't need Cat's negativity and cynicism in her life as she set out to make significant changes to her eating, exercise and overall wellbeing.

If you have a Cat in your life, I'd like you to at least consider how you plan to stay the course while this person tries to throw you off your goals. I'm all for people working things out, so if you can train your Cat not to berate, insult or sabotage by being firm about what you are doing and why, then go for it. Perhaps you and your Cat can find a way to stay friends.

Keep in mind, too, that it's fine for relationships to run their course, and to let go if your Cat is too rooted in her ways to change, or you can see clearly now that such a person was never really your friend. When you do what is best for you you'll know it because your heart will feel lighter and like a whole new space has opened in it.

Tips for Going the Distance

Breaking the addiction to garbage foods and drinks

As you start eating real foods over the next few days, you may experience withdrawals from soda and other sources of sugar, chemicals, salt and fat that is plentiful in garbage foods. Please stick with it. After the first three days or so, you will begin to feel better.

Be patient with yourself as you fight the cravings, and get through the first few days. If you have been a heavy soda drinker, you may want to cut down to one soda every day for one week, and then three sodas a week in week two. Soda is especially addictive, mostly because of the high sugar and caffeine content. From week three on, I'd like you to only drink soda on your cheat day, which we'll go over in a little bit. You are breaking an addiction, just like others break addictions to drugs, cigarettes or alcohol. This is no small thing.

For the first six months or so of making major changes to my diet, and learning to eat smaller portions as well, I used Skinny Cow ice-cream bars and Fiber One brownies like heroin addicts use methadone. If you don't need these daily treats like I did, that's wonderful. But if you do, they can help. If such treats tend to trigger you to eat several, then buy them in the single serving size, or don't have them in the house.

Getting movement in

It's time to begin exercising and sweating now, as sweat releases toxins, and exercise reduces stress. You are becoming healthy, because you are getting all the bad stuff out, and putting the good stuff in. Your body gets the bad stuff out of your body in the form of sweat.

We will go into how to get cardio and strength exercise in detail in Chapter 6. For now, I'd like you to start looking for ways to get movement in for thirty minutes about three to four times per week – with brisk walks or bike riding, on an elliptical or treadmill at your gym, or in a Zumba, yoga or other class.

What to eat in the morning, and what to pack for the day

If you wonder what to eat, start your day with your favorite coffee, tea or low-sugar juice. An egg or two with chicken or turkey bacon or sausage are high in protein, and will fill you for hours; slow-cooked oatmeal topped with fruit and nuts, or a whole grain or sprouted English muffin are great, too.

Once you've had a good breakfast, your next step is to pack a substantial amount of food for the day so that you're not hungry, or tempted to get the wrong food later. I almost always take a big spinach salad with lean meat, Greek yogurt, two pieces of fruit and some nuts.

I cannot stress enough how important it is that you have enough food with you for the day. You do not want to run out of food, and end up staring longingly at chocolate in the vending machine, or wind up at the fast food drive-through. If you'll be gone for two meals, make sure you have two meals with you.

If you eat nutritious foods, stay full throughout the day and get some exercise in a few times a week, you win.

Eat protein with every meal

Eating protein with every meal is so important that if you were to make this one change to you diet, I believe that you would lose weight. When you add protein to every meal, you will feel full. I cover this further in Chapter 4 – Fat Loss for Good, but I want you to get started with this essential tip for being full and well-nourished.

Eating protein helps by boosting the metabolic rate, and reduces appetite because it is so much more filling than fat or carbs.

In one study, obese men who ate a diet consisting of 25 percent protein increased feelings of fullness, and reduced snacking late-night by half. Women also succeeded on the higher protein diet, for when those who participated in the study took in 30 percent of their calories from protein, they ate 441 calories less per day, and lost 11 pounds in 12 weeks....just by adding protein!

Here are some examples of protein to add to your meals: turkey, chicken, ham, beef, cheese (in moderation), almonds, natural peanut or almond butter, eggs and Greek yogurt.

A salad a day

Make a salad topped with protein in the form of egg, lean meat or tofu. The salad provides you with the nutrients you need in a delicious meal. It fills you up and satisfies you, so that you are less likely to eat garbage food. I promise that you will feel invigorated after eating this salad, instead of fatigued from carb-heavy lunches.

I've put kale or spinach on the list of foods for you to buy and eat daily, because dark greens are rich in vitamins and minerals. Iceberg lettuce is simply roughage, and provides no nutrition.

It's also important that you look carefully at nutrition labels before using a salad dressing. Stay away from dressings high in sugar, fat, calories and sodium. I recommend oil and vinegar, or a natural or organic salad dressing.

Top your salad with tomato and avocado slices, sunflower seeds, and a hard-boiled egg and olives, if that's what you like. Dried fruit is okay in moderation, because it is high in sugar. The salad should be delicious, and make you feel satisfied.

Dinner is a lighter meal than breakfast and lunch

Whether you eat dinner at home or out, I recommend that dinner be lighter than lunch, and consist of protein, positive fat and vegetables, with no refined carbs. Bread, pasta and sugar are meant to be consumed in the morning and afternoon in small portions, when we have the chance to burn off the calories.

The heavier meals of your day should be breakfast and lunch. Doesn't it make sense that dinner will be the lightest meal, since you won't be burning many calories after dinner time?

Have a cheat day:

As you combat cravings for your favorite foods each day, write down each craving as it comes up. Then schedule a cheat day once a week when you can have what you are craving. The cheat day will not throw off your weight loss goals unless you eat excessively.

This is not a day to go hog wild, and eat everything in sight. It is a day to enjoy some treats that you've been missing. The great choices you make during the other six days of the week will add up, and the one cheat day will not hurt your progress.

My cheat day last week looked like this: two slices of french toast on multi-grain bread with turkey bacon; rotisserie chicken and Greek yogurt for lunch; an apple and almonds for a snack; and dinner out was a burger with half the bun, half an order of garlic fries, an eight-ounce beer and half a piece of cake.

This was 100 percent better than the way I ate when my weight was much higher; then, I rushed through each meal, sometimes hiding in my car at the side of a fast food joint so that no one would see me indulging. Now, I get to enjoy foods I crave on cheat day openly without shame, while keeping an eye on how to make even the cheat meals a little healthier.

Create a plan for the munchies

Create a plan for the munchies around your specific cravings in a way that allows for you to be satisfied, whether they be for something creamy, salty, sugary or fizzly. Get in the habit of making the healthiest choice available, such as a sweet potato instead of french fries, or a creamy Greek yogurt instead of ice-cream. Each healthy substitution you make is a step away from fat prison.

"Food reveals our connection with the Earth. Each bite contains the life of the sun and the earth…We can see and taste the whole universe in a piece of bread! Contemplating our food for a few seconds before eating, and eating in mindfulness, can bring us much happiness." -Thich Naht Hanh

Chapter 2

A Healthy Body, not a Perfect Body

As I guide you through the habits that lead to health, vitality and a weight that's right for you, keep in mind that this is not about attaining physical perfection.

"Perfection is the enemy of good." Which wise person said this first is unknown. The words are powerful because they bring us to the realization that by aspiring for perfection, we aspire for something unattainable, like a body most of us are never going to have because it isn't real. Our goal is: a healthy body, not a perfect body.

When we hate our bodies because they don't measure up to what we see on the cover of a magazine or in our fancy, tiny-sized neighbor at the grocery store, this mental framework keeps us in a frustrating cycle of never reaching a healthy weight, because 98 percent of us are just not genetically wired to look like a supermodel.

I believe that the best way to handle the issues of our skinny culture is to first be aware of the differences between a real body, and a model's body. A model must often come close to starving herself to wear a small size. The images we see of models are airbrushed and Photo-shopped, and these images do not represent the way that person looks in real life.

The actress Kate Winslet told GQ regarding her digitally-altered image on the magazine's front cover, "The retouching is excessive. I do not look like that, and more importantly, I don't desire to look like that."

Women are not the only ones who are bombarded with messages that we don't measure up. Look at the cover and content of men's fitness and health magazines. The message is: a man has almost no body fat, and eight-pack abs. Even though he is expected to earn a decent living to be a real man, he must have two hours a day to work out to be super buff.

Rocco, my favorite barista, tells me that men have worse pressure to be buff because "it's okay when girls are thicker, but not as much for guys."

Many of my male clients dread even the small amount of belly fat that almost all of us have, and that is inevitable at forty. My guys want to know what they can do to have firm abs and big "mirror muscles" (the arms and chest they can flex in the mirror). I tell them the same thing I tell women—that there is no way to spot reduce body fat, and that if they want killer abs and lots of tone, that big changes to nutrition and time spent working out is required, and that even then, they're going to need dumb genetic luck. Some men are not genetically predisposed to bulk up, especially the long, lean ones, just like many women aren't genetically predisposed to be a size 2.

My message to both guys and girls is to say "who cares," and to strive to be beautiful in your own individual way. The way God created you is just right, and your job is to bring out your individual beauty. The new behaviors around eating and exercise I will show you do lead to a beautiful body. By beautiful, I mean healthy, vibrant and strong, not necessarily ultra-slender.

For the next 90 days, I challenge you to stop looking at fashion magazines. Stop when you find yourself comparing yourself to people who are more petite or buff. It's your original body you have to work with, and it can be beautiful with the right care.

The awareness that our bodies are less than ideal begins early. The origins of body shame often begin when our bodies are first developing, if not earlier.

Between seventh and eighth grade, I became aware of my own body as a jiggling, cumbersome thing, suddenly embarrassing and in the way. As a 13-year-old in the doctor's office for my annual visit, I was shown a chart that told me that based on my height of 5'4", I should weigh 120 pounds, five pounds lighter than my weight at the time. I took this as proof that my body was all wrong. I would like to rip up every weight chart on the face of the earth, because these charts don't take into account individual body composition, frame or bra size.

To make matters worse, my aunt told me that boys didn't want to go out with girls who were five or ten pounds overweight, and always preferred skinny girls. I will tell you that my lovely aunt, who was only trying to save me the pain she thought was ahead for an overweight girl, was wrong. I didn't have any trouble finding a guy to love me, even at my heaviest. And I met the love of my life a few years ago . . . at the gym!

But let's back up, so that I can tell you how I first became heavy. When I hit my mid teens, I began to soothe with comfort food, and hid my developing body under layers of fat. I had taken sex-ed, but didn't know the other facts of life: that because I had a bigger body type than a skinny girl, that I was going to be thick and curvy, and that young women are meant to carry fat around the hips and breasts.

Instead of understanding these things, I believed that I had a freak body. I dug into pizzas, and microwaved macaroni and cheese. I ate my dad's Dove bar stash. Hotdogs, hamburgers and fries were regular lunches. A kid playing sports might have burned all this off, but I was not on any teams. I was shocked to see that my weight was up to 180 when I got on the bathroom scale one summer.

I was 15 at this point, and hated being overweight. I hated wearing jeans that were so tight they hurt my stomach, the way my thighs rubbed together and the way the fat bounced when I ran the bases in gym class. I was so ashamed of my body and the extra belly fat that I carried that I hid my torso under big shirts, and hugged my books to my chest with downcast eyes, praying that no one would see my body.

By junior year of high school, I was listening to all the messages about getting skinny, and thus happy and successful, so I began then what would kick off more than twenty years of on-again/off-again dieting. On my first diet, I stuck to a 800-calorie-a-day regiment, and lost 35 pounds. A photo of me from this time shows what looks like a pale, sickly middle-aged woman. My parents and teachers all applauded me for being thin, even though I was often on the verge of passing out, because my 800 calories per day might consist of a can of Pepsi, fries and a Snickers bar. The dark greens, seeds, vegetables, fruit and protein sources that would have nourished me were absent from my diet.

Our bodies need nutritious fresh food and exercise, not the nutrient-void candy bars, fast food and soda that I was eating in my junior year attempt at skinny. This is what I finally grasped as the weight came off for good 25 after that first crash diet. I had to embrace my original body and love it, with all its imperfections, and completely reject the negative messages that come at all of us about what our bodies should look like. This major shift in my thinking had to happen before the numbers on the scale could get any lower.

Then I had to put nutritious food into my body, and stop giving it garbage. I had to sweat and lift weights to burn fat. I had to erase from my thinking the early messages my teachers and peers sent me early on because "Only skinny people are beautiful, loved and respected" just couldn't work in my life anymore.

I want to show you how to replace all those negative messages with positive words that will direct your behavior toward self-love, and all the benefits that come from this new mindset, including healthy weight.

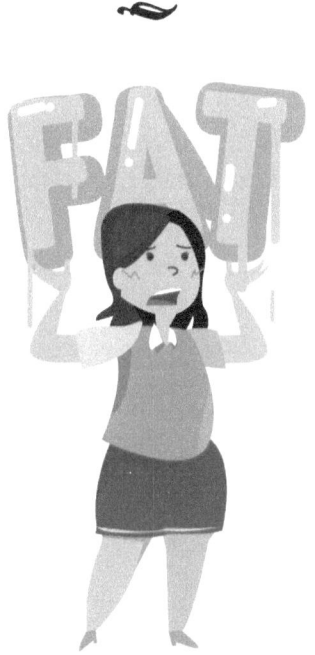

It makes me sad and angry that most of the women and some of the men I know spend time hating their own bodies. Just listen to the people around you talk about themselves. Even women who look slim and stunning say that they feel they are never good enough. How can any of us fully live our lives and be happy if we think that our own bodies are ugly? I've come far from where I used to be when I avoided the bathroom mirror entirely lest I catch a glimpse of my body and hear the words "freak," "ugly" and "cow" resonate in my mind.

Whenever one of my girlfriends complains about the fat on her hips and thighs, I smile knowingly, because I have to fight the fat my body loves to put on my belly. We each have unique bodies that pack protective fatty layers on certain spots. The body puts fat over the organs or on the hips, abdomen, butt or thighs to protect us from stress, disease or potential starvation.

This does not mean that I think it's healthy to be significantly overweight, because carrying around a lot of extra pounds is hard on the body and spirit. For every 25 pounds of extra body weight carried, the heart has to pump to 5,000 miles of additional blood vessels (Western Washington University, 2012). That's a lot of extra work for your heart, and strain on your joints. Every time you take a step, there are four pounds of pressure per one pound of body weight on the knees and ankles.

The way to get rid of that extra fat and attain a leaner, lighter self is through choices made throughout your day, often the choices that seem small but add up, like ordering an iced tea (zero calories) instead of a big, sugary frappuccino (340 calories). When each choice you make around what you put in your mouth comes from self-love, each choice propels you toward greater health.

In addition to what's going in your mouth, you're going to have to look at what's going into your mind, because from your thoughts come action. If you tell yourself that you can't lose weight or you can't exercise, your behavior will reflect what you're telling yourself.

Look at your body and appreciate it, even though it may not look exactly the way you wish it did. Your entire body, every cell in fact, does constant work to make it all happen for you. Tell your body that from this moment on, that you are going to treat it with love and respect. Find at least two things that you like about yourself: beautiful hair, glowing skin, pretty eyes, nice shoulders, whatever qualities you value. When you find yourself criticizing your body, remember what it does for you, and the things you like about it most. In this way, you rewire your thinking.

Here are some examples of things I used to say to myself when I was stuck at 197 pounds, and the messages I replaced them with on my way to being lighter and healthier:

Negative message: My body is ugly.
Loving message: My body works hard for me. I'm finally giving it the care it deserves.

Negative message: I must have pizza! Now!
Loving message: I'll either choose to have 1-2 pieces now with a salad, or I'll plan to have it for lunch later this week.

Negative message: I can't lose weight, and might as well not try.
Loving message: I make choices that result in me being healthier and lighter.

Negative message: I'm too fat and out of shape to go to the gym.
Loving message: People of all body types exercise, and it changes their lives.

Tips for going the distance

Use body fat percentage rather than the scale to help you determine a healthy weight

I believe that body fat percentage shows individual health and body composition more effectively than the scale. Body fat percentage charts are based on age group, and give ranges of healthy numbers to strive for instead of a one-size-fits-all number based on height.

Shift your thinking from trying to reach a low number on the scale to getting into a healthy body fat percentage range for your age group.

To get your body fat percentage, ask the desk staff at your local fitness center or your doctor to measure it for you. Next, go online and look up the acceptable and fit body fat percentage categories for your age group. I advise taking your body fat once a month, and once you reach your goal, settle on a healthy weight range of about 3-5 pounds to maintain.

For instance, an acceptable body fat percentage for me is 27-28 percent. My weight is between 148-152 pounds when I hit a 27-28 percent body fat percentage, so I consider somewhere within these numbers to be a desirable place for myself to land on the scale.

The American Council on Exercise (ACE) breaks it down for us. The ACE considers an acceptable body fat percentage for women to be 25-30 percent; 21-24 percent is considered fit. A man in the fit range would be 14-17 percent body fat; up to 25 percent would be acceptable. These numbers are a good rule of thumb to follow for most of us. High school athletes and those with naturally smaller physiques will probably fall within lower body fat percentages.

You will see your body fat percentage go down, along with your weight, as you incorporate cardio/strength workouts into your life a few times a week, and as you improve your nutrition. Expect great things. They are about to happen!

Chapter 3

Getting Real About What You Eat

The experience of wanting to lose weight, and never being able to pull it off feels like insanity. Seeing the numbers on the scale stay the same or increase when you have tried multiple diets is maddening.

When I began to eat and exercise in a way that resulted in a healthy weight, I did one thing that made all the difference between being stuck in denial about my eating and exercise habits, and finally getting lasting results: I began to track what I was eating.

Without the awareness of what you're eating and drinking on a day-to-day basis, it's nearly impossible to see results on the scale, or the improved vitality that positive nutrition brings.

Track your food so that you see what is going into your mouth in black and white. When I was losing 1-2 pounds per week over about 14 months' time, I used food/fitness tracking apps to log all my food and exercise. Some of my clients swear by their Fitbits.

Using these tools to support your efforts makes it easier to think about how to choose healthy food to meet your weight loss and fitness goals. I encourage you to find a way to track that works for you, whether it be with a website/app, or a notebook and pen.

I have found the Weight Watchers SmartPoints program extremely helpful for many people because it is simple accounting for food. Weight Watchers is a company of people who listen to their customers, and want to always evolve. The SmartPoints program is effective. While Weight Watchers members get a SmartPoints range to shoot for each day along with bonus points for the week, they are rewarded for eating nutritious, protein-rich foods because these foods have less points.

My clients who get results on the scale track their food using whatever way works best for them, so that we can see patterns such as when cravings hit and what healthier substitutions could be made for sugar/fat bombs. We look at their food logs, and can see together what's working, and what needs to be changed in their daily eating.

One of my new clients, Mary Beth, began writing everything down that she ate after our first session together, during which we set a weight loss goal for her of 1-2 pounds per week. Tracking opened her eyes as to how much she was eating, and how many desserts were sneaking their way in.

During her first week, Mary Beth tracked five "fun-sized" candy bars (I always thought that candy bars that size were not big enough to be that much fun!), which called to her from the break room at work every afternoon. I thanked Mary Beth for telling me what was going on so that we could get strategize.

The next week, Mary Beth brought almonds and low-fat cheese sticks to work. These protein snacks filled her, and kept the sugar cravings away (for the most part). She ate one fun-sized candy bar instead of five during the week. On Mary Beth's second weigh in, she had lost three pounds. She told me that the biggest reason for this was that she tracked her food every day.

When you track everything, even the foods you wish you hadn't eaten, you are keeping it real. There is no room to play with denial here. Denial will do whatever it takes to keep you in old behavior.

Without seeing what is happening right in front of you, it's too easy to stay stuck on the scale, stuck in denial and stuck in the patterns that are not serving your goals. In other words, your denial will win and you will be blocked from attaining a healthy weight, liberation from fat prison and happiness.

One of my hardest-working clients, Carrie, has taken 45 pounds of fat off her 5'6" frame so far. In the first couple of months, Carrie would stick to the diet we'd agreed on and then backslide every few weeks. She never hid what was going on during these times. If she ordered a pizza and ate the whole thing, she tracked it.

There was one particular time Carrie and I will never forget. She used good judgment at first, and threw half a pizza away. Yet not too long after, Carrie fetched the box out of the trash and ate the rest. We looked at why she ordered the pizza in the first place: as a quick fix to fill her feelings of loneliness and emptiness, and to provide self-medication for a stressful week.

These kind of days happen, so we need strategies around them. I helped Carrie come up with a pizza strategy for the next time she had cravings: she would keep an organic frozen pizza on hand, and make that instead (360 calories for the whole thing instead of about 2,000 in the take-out pizza).

Do you have a pizza strategy? If it's not pizza that is your downfall, what can you honestly say you dug out of the trash recently?

Right now, I want you to ask yourself what your thoughts and feelings are when you succumb to trigger foods, and eat much more than you had planned on. What emotions seem to overtake and direct your behavior?

Take a pen out, and write down what's going on before you start eating your trigger food next time. Even better, use this as an opportunity to put the trigger food away, and choose something healthier that will fill your craving.

When you write down what is going on in your mind, this will help you see what you are using the food for: to fill loneliness, provide relief from boredom or fulfill a self-defeating prophecy that you are not meant to succeed in becoming healthier and lighter. These are all common reasons why we eat what we shouldn't. Having the reasons why in front of us provide clarity, and help us choose better.

The next important step I want you to take is to think about doing healthy living 95 percent consistently, not 100 percent inconsistently. I believe in doing good eating and exercise habits that work forever, instead of a diet that lasts for two weeks. You are going to eat real foods with room for a treat here and there, instead of embarking on a strict diet that is miserable, and not doable for long.

What I've found works in the long-term is a diet of real food and regular exercise that you can do for life, and that leaves room for get-togethers, weekly treats, and bad days. Without some wiggle room for treats, and a couple of rest days from exercise per week, your new habits will not be sustainable.

What I'm talking about is getting off the crazy merry-go-round of dieting, when we see weight drop off then come back on. This often is the end result of trying to be good 100 percent of the time; you end up being bad, maybe really bad, for several months, and this is when weight comes back on or increases.

Doing 95 percent may sound odd because we are often told to give 100 percent. The problem with giving 100 percent when it comes to eating and exercise is that it's unrealistic, and leads to inevitable failure. What doing 95 percent means is that we eat foods like lean meats, vegetables, Greek yogurt and whole grains 95 percent of the time. Because I know that 5 percent being bad (in moderation) is allowed, I enjoy a kid's size ice-cream cone or piece of pizza so much more than when these kind of foods took up a good part of my diet. We are all going to have slip ups, cravings and bad days. When we do 95 percent, all the good choices add up. The weight comes off, and stays off.

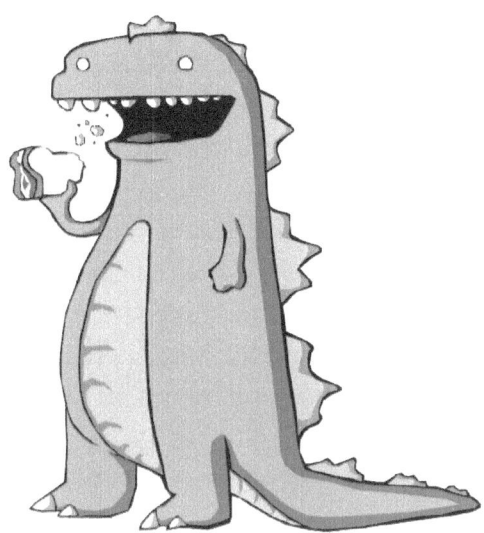

My pizza-loving client, Carrie, inspires me because she sticks with our vision for her as a lighter, healthier person, and knows how to get creative about it. Carrie texted me the other day about another success. Carrie and her son, Samuel, had stopped at Trader Joe's before leaving for a road trip to visit family. The last time they'd taken a road trip, they ate Pringles, Cheetos and Oreos. This time, Carrie decided to stock up on some snack foods that are a lot better for her and her family's health: kale chips, snap peas, organic cookies and seltzer water.

Yes, you read right—cookies. Carrie needed to make positive changes without feeling deprived. The cookies are part of her 5 percent wiggle room for the week (remember, we are looking for a 95 percent success ratio in healthy living). Because Carrie kept her portion down to four cookies over two days of the trip, she didn't throw off her nutrition plan.

If Carrie had hit the road with a bag of veggies and bottled water, she might wind up giving in to her cravings for her favorite super-sized fast food meal. By taking the healthy snacks along, plus the cookies, she saved a boatload of calories, fat and sugar.

While Carrie may not have lost weight the week of her road trip, she didn't gain weight either, which would have been the end result if she had stuck with her former habits. The new way of thinking of healthy living I am introducing you to reinvents the way you may have been taught to think about success and failure. The old way is black and white, and unrealistic. Success is the decision you make today to eat real foods instead of overly processed garbage foods, and to do exercise you enjoy several days each week.

Don't expect perfection. You are human. The difference between you and someone who quits after a few weeks is that you never give up. You keep giving it a shot, until your daily, moment by moment choices feel like the natural thing to do, and you have a healthy, fit body to show for it.

You may be surprised to hear that most of my weight loss clients tell me that they come to like the new habits I'm telling you about, and that the new habits become easier to do consistently than the old habits of swinging through the drive-through or snarfing down half a pizza.

I find the new habits liberating, because there's no guilt or other bad feelings when I eat a piece of pizza, and I delight in each lick of an ice-cream cone, because I have these as special treats instead of part of my regular diet. I view food as something that nourishes my body, not something that makes me feel fat or guilty. When I have my weekly treat day, the foods I once ate quickly and with shame and a sense of defeat are savored openly instead.

When I ate to fill a void of loneliness, to self-medicate during a rough day or just because naughty garbage foods tastes good, I ate quickly, and within two minutes the good feelings were gone. Even if I did enjoy the taste of the food, I had a bloated stomach and world of shame and guilt.

This is a process that takes time for all of us. It took me more than a year to go down from 202 pounds and 39 percent body fat to 155 pounds and 27 percent body fat. Your weight, girth measurements and body fat are going to go down, too.

To get there, you start right now. Not tomorrow or Monday morning. Now. Then you understand this is a daily practice in creating a whole new life mindset, not a quick fix that fails again in a month.

Tips for going the distance

Be aware that readiness to lose weight comes in stages

Don't be surprised if you start, stumble and stop a few times on your way to your healthy weight. The transtheoretical model of behavior change says that people make changes through a series of stages, not all at once.

There is the contemplation state first, during which you recognize that changes need to happen in your eating and exercise habits. This was the phase I was in the night of the big brownie, and it went on for several years before I got to the action phase. Between the contemplation and action phase is the preparation phase, during which you do some reading on healthy living and/or sign up at a gym, taking small steps toward change. The action phase is when you actually start eating healthier foods and getting your work outs in. In maintenance, you have been sustaining your healthy new habits for a few months, and working to ensure you don't backslide. In the termination phase, you are no longer tempted to go back to unhealthy behavior around food. I'm not sure if this has ever happened for me fully, but I can pass a donut or fast food place now without going in!

Confronting the Saboteur

Have you ever gone through a few days of doing a diet, taking all the steps necessary, only to self-sabotage in grand style? My favorite way was to do diet XYZ for about two weeks, then say f* it, order a pizza and breadsticks, and put on a movie at home. I should have put a sign near the couch that said, "Don't bother me, I'm going to be fat." We've all been there. We buy the right foods or diet aids, get the gym membership, then fall into an abyss.

My plan allows for some backsliding, especially at first. We are in this for the long haul, and the difference is that we don't give up. We don't let the backsliding incidents ruin everything. Tomorrow is another day to make the right choices. After all, this is about a new, healthier life in which happiness and vibrancy are the goals. I promise you that the majority of good choices, that 95 percent, will add up. At first, you may find that you are doing 80 percent, not 95 percent. Stay the course. The changes we are talking about take time to do consistently. Being perfect or not at all is not doable long-term.

The other thing that goes on within many of us that interferes with weight loss success is the saboteur. The saboteur is the part of ourselves that tries to ruin our positive efforts toward success by urging us to give up on our goals, and make the wrong choices.

Before I figured out how to eat and exercise effectively, I would set out with the best intentions in many areas of my life. Fortunately, the saboteur didn't interfere when it came to my career, and I was able to win people's trust, work hard for them and make some money along the way. However, when it came to eating and exercise, the saboteur was in control.

I've met other people like this. They are often very successful in their careers. However, when it comes to food and exercise, they feel a lack of control over something as simple as what goes in their mouths.

I was mystified about my own self-sabotaging behavior until I met a life coach, Andrea, in the era of the Big Brownie. I told Andrea how I often changed my eating and exercise to a healthier format, then gave up after a time, and went back to the big dessert portions and fast food I craved. Andrea said that she believed that there was a side of myself, a saboteur, who was ruining my efforts to get slimmer and healthier.

With this realization came an instant sense of peace and calm. I was no longer out of control. I could drive, and the saboteur could talk to me from the backseat.

Last week, my saboteur said that she didn't want to go to the gym. She wanted to just go home, and watch Netflix. Even though it sounded tempting to go home, because it was a cold, icky day, I reminded myself that I was going to make the best choice, one that would involve more effort, but one that would get me toward instead of away from my goals. I drove into the gym parking lot instead of back home, and the minute I went through the doors, I was glad. It felt great to move my body, and sweat. My workout made me feel strong and energized.

The saboteur interferes with decision making when it comes to eating also. The saboteur sends you messages that you may as well just order a pizza or get fast food on the way home from work because you've had a bad day, and making a healthy meal is just too time-consuming.

It's time to identify the saboteur and its destructive intent, then learn how to ignore its messages, and do positive things for yourself instead.

- What are some messages your saboteur gives you when it wants to ruin the positive steps you take toward healthier eating and/or exercise?
- Who is your saboteur? What does s/he look like?
- What can you say to your saboteur when s/he wants to ruin everything?

"It is a shame for a man to grow old without seeing the beauty and strength of which is body is capable." -Socrates

Chapter 4

Fat Loss for Good versus Diet Madness

During my diet failure years, I laid on the couch once with a migraine for three days while I drank only water mixed with tree sap and cayenne pepper. Jen, who was my partner in crime, was on her couch as well with a terrible headache.

For "dessert," we sprayed apple pie-scented potpourri spray into the air, and inhaled as the chemical sweet droplets fell into our faces. Jen and I would have followed the tree sap diet for ten days if we'd done as the diet intended, but we both cracked on the morning of the fourth day. We each lost two pounds of water weight, which we promptly put back on as we restored ourselves with large meals.

When I was losing my weight, I did it eating 1,200-1,500 calories per day. Knowing that I was going to get enough food throughout each day made my new eating habits sustainable. If I had felt deprived and hungry, I wouldn't have been able to stay the course. Still, I had to create a ***calorie deficit*** to lose weight. This means simply that you burn more calories than your body uses. A healthy diet and exercise both factor in to create your calorie deficit. You take in less calories than you were before you started eating healthy, and you burn calories through exercise once your workout routine takes off.

I advise that women not go below 1,200 calories per day on rest days or 1,400 on workout days, and that men take in at least 1,700 on rest days or 2,000 on workout days. You are going to need nourishing food, and calories will be required for your exercise. I call it "positive nutrition." Quality calories that come from foods like lean meats, eggs, tofu, nuts, seeds, fresh fruit and vegetables have a much different effect on your body composition than nutrient-void fast food and other garbage foods.

Remember that to lose one pound per week, you have to burn 3,500 calories, while making sure that you have enough food to feel full. A weight loss goal of one pound per week is appropriate. If you do the healthy habits I'm outlining 95 percent of the time, you can count on keeping those pounds off.

The amount of calories you need every day to function at rest can be calculated by getting your Basal Metabolic Rate. There is an equation for this you can easily look up online. However, because the way in which your body burns calories is based on several factors such as age, and whether your weight has yo-yoed in the past, (if yours has, like mine, then you are more likely to have a harder time losing weight) BMR won't tell you everything. My BMR is 1,348, however I feel hungry when I eat less than around 1,450 calories per day, especially on the days I work out. Having a calorie goal to shoot for helps you stay on your weight loss goals, because calories actually do count. You want those calories to count, to nourish you.

There is a big difference between losing weight in a way that's healthy and stays off, and losing weight in a way that is unhealthy and very likely to come back on, like those two hard-earned pounds of water weight my friend and I lost, then put right back on.

The Center for Disease Control and Prevention reports that *68 percent of people over 20 are either obese or overweight, and that 45 million people are on a diet.* A small percentage of these dieters lose weight while dieting, and an even smaller percentage keep weight off.

The problem with most diets is that they don't take into account the way the body functions while losing weight: muscle versus fat loss; how to ensure that muscle is not depleted during a diet; the way that carbs and protein effect weight; and how to elevate, not hinder, digestion and metabolism.

Positive nutrition isn't about eating only one type of food, or dropping another entirely. There are good carbs like fruits and vegetables, and carbs like bread and cake to be eaten in moderation; there are also good fats like olive oil and nuts, and fats that should only be eaten occasionally like ice-cream. It's about knowing the difference, and eating in a way that nourishes you, and makes you leaner.

Another effective way to account for what you eat, to know how much to eat, is through the Weight Watchers SmartPoints system. "WW" is helping millions of people lose weight permanently with its smartest program yet. I'm in the process of losing my last ten pounds with the help of Weight Watchers, and would recommend it to everyone. At no time do I feel like I'm on a diet that involves deprivation.

When we are "on a diet," we often find that *we feel depleted*, because the diet drinks/shakes or frozen entrees often contain less nutrients than what we actually need.

Positive nutrition is so much more effective than dieting. Dieting involves deprivation, hunger and often eating food that tastes like cardboard. After a few days or weeks of this, the normal reaction for most of us is to give up.

Another reason I prefer "positive nutrition" over "diet" is because of all the connotations of the D word. The D word makes me think of my earliest associations with weight loss attempts: the Tab soda, and frozen diet dinners that my Aunt V. had in the fridge/freezer. About once a year, these items replaced the regular food in Aunt V's 'fridge. It always ended the same way, with Aunt V. digging into a lemon meringue pie then berating herself.

Aunt V. was big-boned and sturdy, not petite like my mom. I didn't understand why V. was disgusted by her body, so much that she was willing to make herself miserable dieting. I loved my aunt for many reasons, especially her wit, and sarcastic sense of humor.

Aunt V. died at the age of 98. I regret that this intelligent, independent-minded woman spent seventy years or so berating herself for being unable to lose weight.

Aunt V. thought that being lighter was a matter of either almost starving herself while existing on unpleasant foods, or getting to eat the foods she loved at the cost of being overweight.

With a positive nutrition plan, I want you to lose fat instead of water and muscle. Since fat takes up a lot of space, that 1-2 pounds that comes off every week is going to **look** like progress, because when you lose a pound of fat, that's a lot of *space reduction* in inches off your body.

I can remember losing thirty pounds in the first ten weeks of work with my own fitness coach. Ten pounds didn't sound like much after all the sweat and willpower I put forth during those ten weeks. My wise coach pointed out that I had also lost *17 inches*, most of which came off my butt, stomach, hips and chest-- the places where I wanted to lose fat most.

I couldn't have lost those 17 inches without cardio and strength work, because the exercise changed my body composition from fatty to muscular. I burned off thirty more inches over the course of several more months of taking on the healthy eating and exercise habits I live by today.

Here's how exercise makes all the difference: it fires up the metabolism for 36 hours following a workout. Strength training with weights, resistance bands or body weight exercises force your body to burn fat instead of muscle. (See Chapter 6, Real Workouts for Real People to learn more.) *Consistent exercise is essential.*

I believe in setting *weekly weight loss goals* instead of a specific weight to arrive at. This approach sets you up for success, not failure for a couple of reasons:

- ✓ Having a weekly goal feels like something that can actually happen, instead of a mammoth goal such as "I want to lose forty pounds."
- ✓ It's impossible to determine your ideal weight until you experience what you feel like, and look like, at lighter weight ranges.

I've found through my own experience losing significant weight and helping my clients do the same, that setting weekly goals around losing 1-2 pounds is the way to lasting success. On those challenging weeks when weight loss is slower, I want you to **celebrate the small victories**. These weeks will happen. While I was losing my weight, sometimes on a week when I had really worked hard, I saw *no pounds lost*, but then I saw *a bigger loss the following week*. Other times, the scale showed no weight loss or even a gain of a pound because I had enjoyed more weekly treats than usual, or I had been at a special event. This is going to be a process of changing your life, not just a short-term goal for the New Year.

Tips for Going the Distance

Read every food label

Read the food labels as you cook at home, or grab snacks off the shelves. If a food has more than 16 grams of sugar per serving, ask yourself whether you need it, and consider that it won't help you meet your weight loss goals. If you see **high fructose corn syrup** on the label, *don't* put it in your mouth. High fructose corn syrup triggers the same cycle of cravings that sugar does, and *wreaks havoc* on the body's ability to process glucose.

Have a special treat 1-2 times a week

Getting to have an occasional treat means the difference between feeling locked into a diet, and doing *positive nutrition* with allowances for what you *crave* now and then. When you can look forward to your favorite treats once in a while, it's easy to stay the course. Do watch your portions when you enjoy your treat. Have a couple slices of pizza (only one if it's deep dish) with a salad, two cookies instead of a whole row, a half cup or kids size ice-cream scoop, and make sure that slice of pie or cake doesn't take up half the plate. Better yet, share the slice—so much more fun!

Look for the healthiest version of what you crave, for instance organic ice-cream or desserts instead of the run-of-the-mill stuff. This doesn't mean that organic desserts aren't loaded with calories, sugar and fat, so read your food labels.

Eat out smart

We can still eat out at restaurants, and stick with our goals, although I would recommend that you eat out only occasionally because of the sugar, fat and salt that most places add to their food to make it taste great.

A good strategy is looking at the restaurant's menu online before going and deciding what you are going to order before you arrive. Next, make selections from the menu that include more protein and less carbs.

Ask the waiter to take the bread basket away, or split one piece with your dining companion. Ask for vegetables instead of fries, or get a sweet potato if that's an option. If the idea of eating out no more than once in a while sounds boring, or having a dessert and/or alcoholic drink only once a week sounds boring, keep your goals in mind. Is fitting into a smaller size jeans boring? Is liking your body instead of hating it boring? Is going to a wedding in a dress, and being complimented and admired boring? Is feeling confident in your bathing suit boring?

Weigh in once a week, not every day

I don't advise weighing in more than once a week, otherwise getting on the scale can become an obsessive habit. Also, weight can fluctuate throughout the day, so I recommend weighing in in the morning, the same day each week, and on the same scale so that there are no discrepancies.

You are going to reach your healthy weight without pain or deprivation. I know you don't believe me. It's so hard to, because we have been disappointed so many times. But you can believe me, because *I have been exactly where you are right now.*

You can expect good things to happen when you incorporate positive nutrition and exercise into your life. Most of all, you can expect to feel and look better. It's time to get off the merry-go-round of diet failure, and walk on the ground with both feet, each step moving you toward your healthy weight, and your lighter, happier self.

"Life expands or contracts in proportion to one's courage." -Anis Nin

Chapter 5

Taking Back your Power
One Forkful at a Time

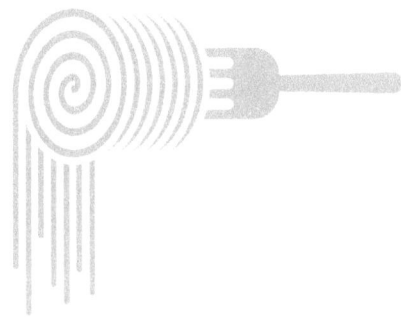

Eating at my former favorite Italian chain restaurant used to make me feel that I was possibly a human with the belly of a whale. No matter how much food I put into my mouth, there was room for more. First came the unlimited salad and breadsticks. Two plates of cheesy salad and several breadsticks (or 700 calories) later, my pasta dish arrived (1,200 calories with the soda).

I was technically full by the time the main course was set in front of me, meaning that my body was telling me there was no room for more food in my stomach, but looking at that fettuccini alfredo, another part of me said I'd be crazy not to dig in.

By the end of the meal, I considered how much food I'd just eaten, and wondered why I wasn't even sure if I was full. About a half hour later, the cramps set in, and my stomach pressed painfully against my waistband. I ended up in the bathroom for an hour, sure that I was having a heart attack at the age of 25. My best girlfriend wanted to call 911, but I assured her that I would be okay.

I hated myself for once again overeating, while mystified by how all that food fit inside my fist-sized tummy. After a couple more decades of research, I learned that I didn't have a whale's stomach, and that what happened to me was happening to millions of people: high-carb restaurant meals actually trick us into thinking that we're still hungry.

We are brought mammoth-sized portions, and we want to clean our plates. We are tricked by the food itself into thinking we're still hungry, then we hate ourselves for eating so much. And so it goes.

It would be easy to conclude from here that it's the food's fault that we overeat, not our own, but we don't get off that easy. We can choose to eat half of a portion, order something healthy and to avoid the restaurants most of the time. We can choose to ask for the grilled option instead of deep fried. We have options, and each choice effects our health, size and ultimately how we feel about ourselves.

The first thing you can do when you're served a large portion is to ask for the to-go box and a bag to put it in, then put half the food into it the minute it's served. Put this bag in the back seat of your car for the ride home, so that you're not tempted to nibble on the way home. Save it for a meal the next day.

The first few times I started taking half of my entrée to go at restaurants, I snuck some of the food out of the box on the drive home. Next, I graduated to getting the leftovers home and into the fridge, but ate it later the same day, sometimes within an hour of arriving home. Next, the food made it until the next meal. Finally, I was capable of saving the food for the next day's lunch. It took me at least an entire year to get from the old way of acting to the new way, because food addiction is very powerful.

If I had given up on the process, and listened to negative inner messages about how pathetic I was, as I stumbled along the path to success, I would have never made it. Remind yourself that you are making changes that will last forever. Breaking lifelong habits is no small thing.

Next, check in with yourself as you eat for signs of fullness. When you eat slowly, you give yourself a chance for your brain to register a chemical message from your body that you're full (It takes 20 minutes). You may notice that feelings of fullness increase after your meal; this is because the levels of the fullness hormone (called leptin) continue to rise for up to half an hour after you take your last bite.

You are going to need a reset so that you can relearn how to feel hungry and full again. The way to do this starts with tuning into the way your body feels. Get back in touch with hungry/full sensations by allowing yourself to feel hungry and then giving yourself time to feel full. This is one of the best things you can do for your health; it means the difference between stuffing yourself and feeling sick, or enjoying food while respecting your body.

Relearning how to tell when you are hungry and need to eat, and breaking patterns of eating out of habit or for emotional reasons is going to take time and practice. It will be a process of returning to your body's natural rhythms. The first step is to commit to an attitude of patience with yourself, because just like with weight loss, we can't expect an entire journey of forward progress to happen in a day.

Between the addictive stuff that's in our food, enormous portion sizes and the impulses to use food to socialize or self-soothe, it's very easy to lose touch with our bodies' own messages about when they are hungry and when they are full.

Let's talk more about allowing ourselves to feel hungry before eating, and being attuned for genuine hunger pangs. Allow yourself to become aware of what hunger feels like. Before you eat next today, wait for your stomach to signal to your brain that you're hungry. This may require eating at a time that is unusual, or that requires you putting yourself and your need to eat before work or other people. The work, and the other people you care for can hold on for a few minutes while you satisfy your hunger with nourishing foods. Eat and drink slowly, enjoying each bite.

Waiting to eat until you're hungry will get easier with practice every day. It will feel like you are respecting your body, instead of letting your mind trick you into eating when you don't need food. If you have stomach issues, you may find that these will diminish as you pay attention to when your body actually needs fuel, and learn to eat at that time.

Feeling full is trickier than feeling hungry

It's hard to know when we're full. The meals served in restaurants are usually 2-8 portion sizes larger than what the USDA recommends.

Keep in mind that the stomach is the size of your fist. Isn't it interesting how big the stomach can stretch to accommodate mammoth portions? Obviously, this isn't good for us. Remember how bad it feels to be overly full, and how bad that you will feel long after the meal has ended.

Combat the old habits of overeating with mindfulness as you get through your meal. Once you are about three-quarter of the way through, ask yourself if you feel full, or if you wish to continue eating. Either answer is fine, *but you want to ask it.*

As you practice checking in with yourself for feelings of fullness, you will discover how much food your body needs, and be able to stop eating at *your* best time.

You've probably noticed that cravings for certain foods feel overwhelming, as though you can't control them. This was my relationship with pasta and pizza for the longest time. It felt like I could chow down forever.

There is an explanation for this: sugar and bread create cravings for more of the same. When carbs and sugar are eaten without protein, the body craves more carbs and sugar. When protein is present along with carbs and sugar, it provides a sense of fullness and absorbs some of the sugar before it can hit your bloodstream, triggering a glucose/insulin release cycle that results in cravings for more sugar. A serving of protein added to a meal or snack helps the body by blocking the impact of carbs/sugar on the blood sugar, which triggers insulin release, which increases the cravings for more carbs/sugar.

Adding protein to every meal is the best way to feel full. Greek yogurt or cottage cheese are great choices. One or two eggs with turkey bacon or sausage for breakfast is another way. Chicken, other lean meat or tofu adds protein to a salad, and makes the meal more substantial.

I'm not anti-carb. I believe that carbs in the form of fruits, vegetables and whole grain bread, rice and pasta in moderation provide essential nutrition.

If you want multi-grain toast or an English muffin for breakfast, make sure you are eating protein along with it. The carbohydrates will have a completely different effect than when they are eaten alone.

When you eat carbs/sugar without protein, they create a buzz for about 30 minutes, and then become a drag on the body; fatigue sets in. So you drink more coffee or soda to stay alert, and by noon you are craving more carbs/sugar. Those early morning carbs/sugar have set you up for cravings!

We are conditioned to believe that less food is better. Most people wouldn't think that adding an egg and/or turkey or chicken sausage to the same breakfast would lead to weight loss, but it does, because you feel full. And without triggering carb/sugar cravings, you are a lot less likely to eat food that you don't need.

Now that you understand the facts about how carbs/sugar effect you, it will be easier for you to avoid foods high in carbs/sugar, except as an occasional treat. When you do eat carbs /sugary foods, combine them with protein to avoid downward spiraling and out-of-control eating.

The American Society of Addiction Medicine defines addiction as characterized by "inability to consistently abstain, impairment in behavioral control, craving, and diminished recognition of significant problems with one's behaviors and interpersonal relationships." Food addiction is as real as alcoholism and drug addiction. It's like any other addiction, in that it grips you, and makes you feel like you have *no control* over your behavior.

Food addiction just doesn't get much press because when someone dies because of food addiction, it's a slow process. People don't often die suddenly from food overdoses. They die from diseases such as diabetes, heart disease or cancer (correlated with unhealthy eating and overeating).

I used food to make myself feel better from the time I was a teenager on, so I can completely understand how strong food addiction is. My clients discuss the same feelings of loss of control over their eating when cravings or stress overwhelm them. Even we personal fitness trainers (some of us were overweight at various points in our lives) have our moments.

My friend and fellow coach, Big D, tells that he has been off his game with food and exercise. Big D said that he used to buy a bag of cookies, take a few out of the bag and throw away the rest, but lately he feels a loss of control over his behavior and ends up eating the whole bag, then hating himself later for allowing himself to lose control.

Big D lost twenty pounds last year, and has gained five back because of his recent binges and lack of exercise. He told me this on his way to teach a group exercise class, where I'm sure none of his students had any idea that he had eaten a bag of cookies recently. It's easy to think that others don't have struggles, especially an exercise leader. But everyone does.

I told Big D to see himself the way I do, and his students do: as a strong, fit, compassionate man who motivates others. Big D just temporarily lost sight of his true self; he's down on himself, so he fulfills his self-prophecy of being unworthy by binging on garbage foods. I trust that he will get through this phase, and return to his regular good habits.

When I was significantly overweight, these are the things I said to myself to rationalize my choice to eat fast food:

> I'll start taking diet pills tomorrow
> I'm hungry, and too tired to make food at home
> Today was hard; this is the best I can do given how hard this day was
> This food will taste good, and make me feel better
> I can't control my cravings, so I might as well give in

Once I got my bag of greasy, nutrient-deficient fast food, I pulled over to a parking space, and was done eating in five minutes or less. Serotonin flooded my system and lifted my mood, because *that's what fast food does.* When I climbed into bed at night, I blocked out thoughts that I had ruined my good intentions once again to eat better, and that I was too smart to behave like this, that I was still sixty pounds overweight and unhappy with my body.

Think carefully about why you put garbage foods in your mouth, **what is going through your mind when you overeat** or choose to eat garbage food.

Stop yourself the next time you want to dig into your favorite garbage foods (that bag of cookies, greasy burger, fries, chips, soda or pizza).

Remind yourself that you can choose to have a healthy snack like fruit and almonds instead, and that you will make a nutritious meal at home. When you stop the anxious thoughts you are having before you buy the garbage food and dig in, you can choose better, and with each choice, affect your health and size.

There will be occasions when your stress or cravings are so overwhelming that you may feel unable to stop yourself from eating garbage foods.

When this happens:

> ➢ Ask yourself how to improve the situation.
> ➢ Can you order broccoli as a side dish instead of fries?
> ➢ Can you split a dessert, or throw half the dessert away?

Making these choices while enjoying your bad meal or snack leaves you with a feeling of satisfaction about improving the situation. Then *forgive yourself*, and let the occasional slip-ups go.

Stress eating, or emotional eating, occurs when the primal part of our brains decides to self-soothe by consuming fat, sugar and salt and grooving on the good chemicals released when comforts foods are taken in. Fat, sugar and salt makes the food taste good, and it makes you feel good temporarily. It makes sense that you crave fries, macaroni and cheese, ice-cream and candy when you feel stressed out. Because you want to arrive at a healthy weight, your primal brain simply needs your higher brain to come to the rescue, and take over decision making about what you are going to put in your mouth during stressful times.

Instead of stress eating, try these ideas instead:

> ➢ Drink water
> ➢ Munch on protein like nuts and cheese, not carbs/sugar

➢ Exercise
➢ Get a massage
➢ Take a bubble bath

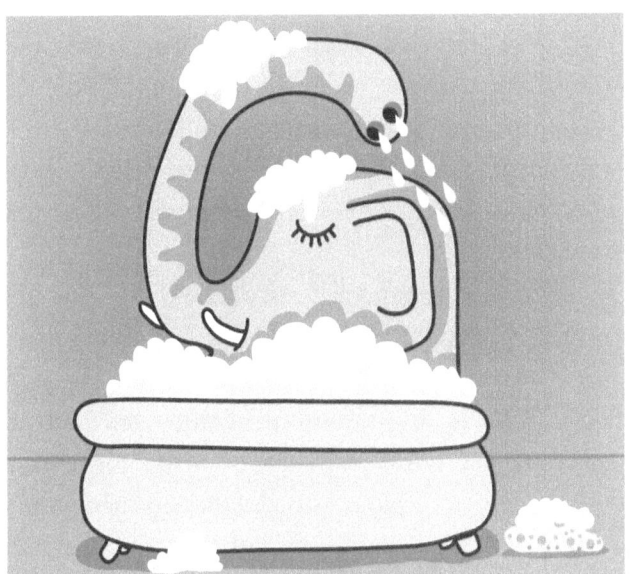

The other day, I passed a fast food restaurant, and thought of how good their fries were. I was hungry, and had about a twenty-minute-long commute left until I got home, where there was a salmon salad and yogurt waiting for me. The fries sounded good, but I chose to go home and eat the healthy dinner, because these foods would taste good while providing more nutrition than the fries. I reasoned that if I still craved fries by the next day, I'd make sweet potato fries at home. They taste even better than fast food fries, and being a super food, are packed with nutrients.

Whenever I want to make a bad choice like eating fries, I remind myself of *what it felt like to be fifty pounds plus heavier*, how my knees and ankles hurt when I walked, and how out of breath I was when I ran the track. Worst of all was *how I felt about my body*, and all the frustration and feelings of failure.

As good as it feels to order from the fast food drive through, and then eat it and feel blissed out for three minutes, **feeling healthy and fit every day feels much better**! Let that be your motivation.

There are days when the thought of having your favorite garbage foods will be very tempting. People don't just do emotional eating when they've had a bad day, although we are especially susceptible then, but when there are simply overpowering cravings for fat, sugar or salt. At these times, places like the fast food drive-through, donut shop, or wherever it is that sells your trigger foods, will have what may feel like a magnetic pull.

This is the time to be especially smart, and vigilant. In the past, when you weren't aware of the importance of making good choices moment by moment, you may have gone to your trigger places as though hypnotized, feeling almost as though you had no choice. When I was in the first few months of embracing positive nutrition, *I had to take another route home* so that I won't even pass the fast food joints that were my trigger places. I thought of other, healthier options that I could have, and went with one of those.

Keep focused, and ask yourself with every meal and snack if you are taking yourself toward or away from your healthy weight goal.

Again, *having enough healthy food with you* so that you're not tempted with the wrong choices is going to set you up for success. When you're full from nutritious food, there is a lot less chance you will be hungry, and craving garbage food.

Tips for going the distance

Have an accountability buddy

Having a friend to call on when you are in the grips of cravings and the desire to fall into emotional eating is essential. I can remember texting my trainer or friend when I passed fast food on the way home from work, or was confronted with a box of ice-cream bars while house sitting. These friends serve as a support system as you break your addiction to the garbage food you have used to soothe hurt feelings, frustration and loneliness for years.

As you learn to eat healthy and kick garbage food out of your life, it will get easier and easier to make better choices. The presence of your support system can make the difference between backsliding or continuing on the right path.

Eat breakfast

Breakfast is very important for setting your metabolism for the day, so I'm going to recommend that you eat something in the morning, even if it's something small. The ideal situation is to wait until you are hungry before eating, so *if you're not hungry* before you leave the house in the morning, take something with you, and eat it when you're ready.

Lunch and dinner

I recommend that lunch be a bigger meal than dinner. This makes sense, since most of us burn more calories in the middle of the day, and less in the evening.

The most loving man in the world packs my lunch every day, so I have protein sources such as turkey slices and cheese, a couple pieces of fruit, almonds and a Greek yogurt. He also makes a delicious dinner for both of us in the evening—a dark, leafy green salad with tomatoes, avocado, seeds and olives, a lean meat or fish, roasted vegetables, and Greek yogurt or fresh fruit for dessert.

Eat what you find to be delicious for your meals and snacks. Food is meant to be enjoyed, and preferences are individual, so create your own version of meals that are predominantly vegetables and protein, and season them to your own taste.

Eating mindfully is life changing. Every time you eat now, you are aware of the food as a source of nourishment, and an investment in your health. The days of eating unhealthy food for the wrong reasons – anxiety, boredom, stress or not knowing what else to do -- are over, and with this important change you are free from fat prison because ***the self-sabotage is over.***

Chapter 6

Workouts that Work

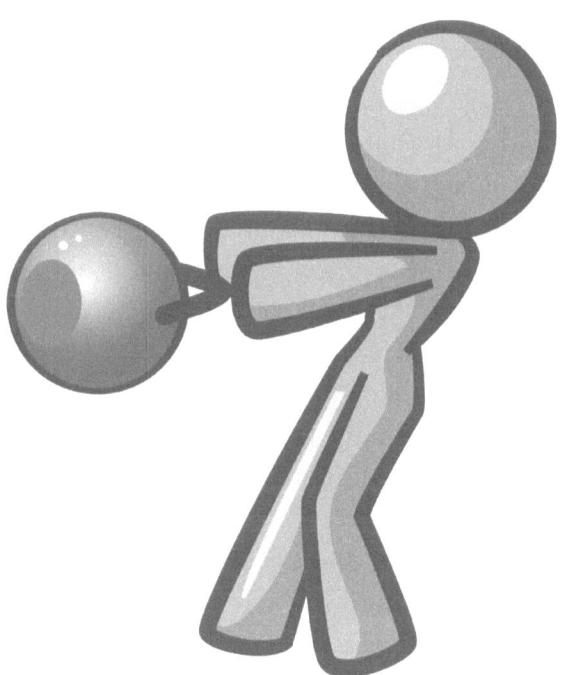

When I ask my clients and the other people I care about to break down the hours of a typical day, we find that some are sitting much of the time. They are fatigued, and many suffer from back pain. These are the common effects of excessive computer use and immobility.

This is not normal or healthy for humans, yet it's the way many people are living.

Our bodies are not designed for inactivity, yet the exercise that makes the body feel so good just doesn't find its way into the day for about 80 percent of people.

According to a 2012 study by the Mayo Clinic, 50 to 70 percent of people spend six or more hours sitting per day, and 20 to 35 percent spend four or more hours a day watching TV. Only 20 percent of people met the weekly Physical Activity Guidelines for both aerobic and muscle-strengthening activity of 150 minutes of cardio activity, and two strength workouts (The Centers for Disease Control and Prevention, 2013).

Companies that care about employees' health include a gym or basketball court onsite, but many businesses do not, so their workers spend hours cramped in a chair.

Consistent exercise means the difference between feeling strong, toned and energetic, or depleted, fatigued and flabby. You want the benefits of exercise: a leaner physique, muscle tone, faster metabolism, fat loss, a stronger heart, stronger bones, stress release, better sleep, more flexibility, higher brain function and greater self-confidence.

Make exercise an almost daily priority, because when you are sedentary, you are not healthy, and if you are not healthy, you will inevitably reach a point where you cannot function. Consistency is everything. When you get your exercise in week after week, you are also less likely to eat poorly.

Humans are not meant to begin a process of decay and atrophy at age forty, or even seventy. People who exercise several times a week enjoy a much better quality of life in midlife and beyond. Those who do not exercise tend to decline over a period of 10-15 years, while the steady exercisers are at the gym feeling great until the very end. Your body wants to be fit and well. It needs a few workouts every week to make that happen.

The human body begins a slow process of breakdown and atrophy beginning in our mid to late twenties. Exercise is truly the fountain of youth. Your muscles and bones get old without exercise. You lose your balance and coordination without it.

My oldest client, Casey, is eighty years old and one of the fittest people I've ever met. He works out three times a week, and skis regularly. Whenever I see Casey, I watch in admiration as he jumps onto a Bosu ball with the agility of a puma, or performs a tough strength-building exercise known as a clean and jerk with a fifty-pound barbell. This exceptional man is building the strength, agility and coordination that usually decline with age.

Exercise should not be a grueling part of the day that you can't wait to get over with. Exercise should be your time, a pause in your busy day where you get to feel better and bring awareness to the importance of caring for your own body.

During extraordinarily busy phases of life, if one workout a week is what you can do, it's infinitely better than nothing and will make the challenges you are facing feel more manageable. Once the chaos lets up, you can return to meeting your goals of several exercise sessions per week.

If you don't get in your workout one day, you get it in the next, until your almost daily exercise goal feels like the new normal.

Before I go into how to get a fun, efficient workout, I have to tell you that without positive nutrition, the body has no chance of attaining a healthy weight. Don't expect to overeat, and burn it all off at the gym. Your body just can't burn off a 1,200-calorie fast food meal of burger, fries and Coke, even during most high intensity workouts.

Sure, there are high school athletes who can stay at a low body fat percentage even while eating whatever they'd like, or that one relative who always has dessert and wears a size 6. These people are exceptions. *For most of us*, a diet of fast food and other overly processed food results in low energy, unhealthy body fat percentage, and skin and hair that doesn't look its best.

At the same time, if both cardio and strength exercise are not present while you are embracing positive nutrition, your heart does not get the exercise it needs during cardio, and without weight-bearing exercise, the body dips into muscle for weight loss instead of burning fat, because the body likes to hang on to cushiony, protective fat.

The body requires healthy protein and carb combinations to perform well during a workout, and without the right nutrients cannot perform at his best. Fast food meals and other garbage foods are nutritionally void, and cannot sustain you through a workout.

I have seen clients become light-headed during exercise when they were not eating well. Keep fruit, nuts or a low-fat cheese stick on hand in your gym locker, in case you need fuel before, during or after a workout. A snack or meal eaten within 45 minutes of a hard workout has been shown to help muscles recover significantly, and this means less soreness and fatigue the next day.

For exercise to happen regularly, it has to fit easily into your daily life. In the same way that positive nutrition must fit right in by keeping your fridge, cabinets and glove compartment filled with the right foods, you must set your environment up so that exercise fits in, too.

This could mean finding a gym that's near your home or work, setting up a space in your home or garage to work out, or getting outside for brisk walks, jog/walk intervals or biking, followed by bodyweight drills like push-ups, squats, lunges, sit-ups and ab exercises.

My workouts include a combination of gym, home and outdoor workouts, because I find that having a variety of exercises and places to exercise breaks up the boredom, and is much more effective at keeping me in shape.

As long as you are moving and sweating and not doing the same exercise every single day, I'm for it. I emphasize mixing up your routine because the body can easily acclimate to one exercise, and not make progress as a result.

Exercise that is motivating for you may not be motivating for me. Zumba isn't my favorite class, but I'm glad it's fun for so many other people. There are many options for cardio: biking, brisk walking, dancing or swimming, which are more fun than pedaling away on a stationary bike or elliptical day after day.

When I didn't feel like getting on a cardio machine at the gym recently, I walked up and down five flights of stairs with a weight, ran around the racquetball court hitting the ball for ten minutes, then got my strength work in with kettlebells. The next day, I felt like putting on my headphones, and getting on the elliptical. *We have options.*

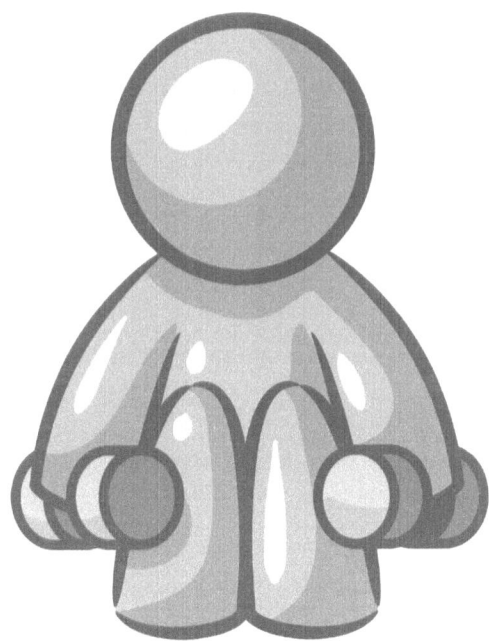

Now I'd like to give you the nuts and bolts of exercise—what to do, and how to do it. One: the first part of your workout should always be cardio. Cardio activity is any movement that increases your heart rate to 60-80 percent of your maximum. This is where effective workouts happen. Whatever movement gets your blood pumping counts as cardio. I only like workouts that are fun for you. I don't care if it's cartwheels, Zumba or skipping, as long as you're doing something in your heart rate range or cardio zone.

The formula used to figure out where your cardio zone is: Subtract your age from 220. Take 60-80 percent of that number. This is your cardio zone. For example, if you're 30 years old, your cardio zone will be 114-152 beats per minute (bpm). If you're 50, it will be 102-136 bpm. Most gyms have machines with sensors for taking your heart rate, and heart rates monitors are sold online.

You'll notice that once you're exercising in your cardio zone, that this where you sweat. Sweating is great because it means that you are working out hard enough to get your heart conditioned. When you sweat, your body releases toxins, too. When I say 'sweat,' I mean that beads of perspiration should form on your body, and that your workout clothes should get a little damp. If you don't like to sweat because there's no time for a shower, try taking some wipes along.

Whatever you do for cardio, go at a pace that is challenging, while sustainable. If you experience joint pain or shortness of breath, stop and recover, or consult with your doctor.

Cardio must also be the first step in every workout, because *muscles must be warm for safe strength training*. When muscles are warm, they are prepared to train. Cold muscles that have not been warmed up with cardio exercise are not ready to take on strength training.

Please be sure to fit in at least ten minutes of cardio activity before you use resistance bands, weights or your own body weight for strength training. Ten minutes is the minimum. I recommend thirty minutes of cardio per session, especially for people with weight loss as a goal.

Getting weight bearing exercise will be the second part of your workout 2-3 times per week. When we talk about weight lifting, if you feel intimidated or squeamish, you're not alone. Some female clients tell me that they have avoided weight lifting in the past because they worried that they would bulk up and gain, not lose weight.

Let me assure you that this is a misconception. *Until I lifted weight, I couldn't seem to lose the fat.* Once I added two or three strength training sessions per week to my workouts, the pounds began dropping. While the pounds were coming off at a pace of 1-2 pounds per week, my body composition was changing rapidly as my body became smaller.

When you exercise consistently and include strength training 2-3 times per week while eating nutritious food, your body will have no choice but to burn fat off.

I can't emphasize enough how important it is that you get both cardio and strength training into your life. Strength exercises can be performed with free weights, kettlebells, resistance bands or body weight. I recommend that you work with a trainer so that you can learn the correct form for each exercise. I would hate to give you a list of exercises to do, only to have you hurt yourself because I'm not there to show you how to perform them the right way.

Joining a fitness facility is an excellent way to get exercise and community into your life. When choosing one, make sure that it's not only a place that's conveniently located, but that it's a place where you feel that the staff really care about you and your health.

The personal trainers should be certified as such, and not just salespeople who say they are personal trainers. Examples of credible places that certify trainers include: AFAA, ACE, ACSM, SCW and NASM.

Once you have bought your membership, the next step is to get an orientation to the fitness center with a coach. This will be more comprehensive than the tour you receive before you join.

During the orientation, the coach will show you how to get a cardio workout using the treadmill, elliptical, bike, etc. and a strength workout using upper and lower body weight machines. Once you have used these machines for a few weeks, I encourage you to consider hiring a personal trainer. Good trainers have an encyclopedia of exercises to draw from and teach. If you're on a budget, simply sign up for a small package of personal training sessions, and meet with your trainer once a week for a month. Take notes during the session, or ask your trainer to email you the workout. This way, you have a record of what you learned, and can do the workouts on your own.

I also recommend adding a group class once or twice a week; the classes beat the boredom of the machines and increase the quality of your workouts. Here are some of the classes on my gym's schedule: Cycling, Boot Camp, Kickboxing, Aqua Aerobics, and Body Pump. I'm sure that at least one of these classes sounds like one you'd like to explore. Even as a trainer who enjoys exercise, I find that I work out harder when I'm surrounded by others who are sweating and having fun. Classes such as Boot Camp or Body Pump may sound a little intimidating, and images of super buff people with little body fat may come to mind. In the Boot Camp class at my gym, we have a grandmother who can probably outrun me, and Tricia, aka "the beast." Tricia has a larger body type, however she brings it 100 percent and is super strong. She lost eighty pounds in the past year through cleaning up her eating and getting steady workouts in on the Stairmaster, plus Boot Camp.

So don't be afraid of not fitting in when you show up for your first class. Introduce yourself to the instructor beforehand, and tell him that you're new. The instructor should help make sure your form is correct, and provide modifications for exercises that may take time to build up to. Just show up, and bring your work ethic and willingness. When you do that, you can't fail!

Tips for going the distance

Home workouts for those days when you can't (or don't want to) get to the gym

You may not have a stationary bike or other piece of equipment at home, but you can still get your cardio in with a brisk walk, biking or jog/walk intervals. There are also workout videos on Amazon to buy or rent.

The following intense cardio exercises will also get you moving and sweating: jumping jacks, burpees, mountain climbers, jump rope and windmills. Do 30 seconds of each exercise, then work your way up to 60 seconds of each. These exercises will warm you up in 5-10 minutes, but they are intense, so you'll probably want to start with something such as brisk walking if you are new to exercise.

Once you've gotten your cardio, you can move into strength training with a set of dumbbells, kettlebells or good old-fashioned bodyweight exercises. I got into the best shape of my life doing push-ups, squats and planks.

A 15-minute workout is infinitely better than no workout

There are different schools of thought regarding the best quantity of time to spend working out. I think that for most of us, 30-45 minutes total is a good goal. If you have 60 minutes to devote to exercise, that's great, but you can still get everything you need out of a 30-minute workout.

What's most important is getting your workout in, so if you have 15 minutes, then use that time to get it done. The short workout means the difference between being consistent on a busy day, and not making time to move. You may be surprised by how good 15 minutes of exercise makes you feel.

Stretching: Do it

Ask your trainer how to stretch the muscles you have been using during strength training. Learn them, and spend just a minute or two throughout your workout stretching, or save stretches until the end. Stretching is important because it allows the muscles to expand after contracting during strength training. Stretching prevents tight, sore muscles the next day. It's something you don't want to skip.

Plan your workout around your day

Each day is not the same. One day you may have to go downtown for a conference, and will have to make some good choices at the lunch buffet. Since the conference is at a hotel, maybe you wear workout clothes under your dressy attire, and bring sneakers along, so that you can get in a workout or a brisk walk on your lunch hour, or after work.

Another day the winter temperatures may be sub-zero, and you'd do anything to get home for the night. That's okay. But do it only with the vow that you will get your Plan B home workout in.

When your body is running optimally on healthy foods, and getting the cardio and strength training it needs to be its best, you just feel good, not just physically. Workouts help release stress; plus. Feeling stronger makes you a lot more empowered to deal with life's challenges.

Working out when you are larger

If normal weight or skinny folks only knew how hard it is to get around the track with 50 pounds plus of extra weight, there would be a lot more respect and compassion for the heavier people who start this journey.

Most often, I start my larger clients out on the bike. This way, they can get their cardio in without any pressure on the joints. Aqua classes are also a great fit, where a larger person can feel lighter in the water, while still getting in a great workout. When I was getting certified as an aqua instructor last year, I learned that moving in the pool burns many more calories per half hour than on the treadmill. For those of us with tweaky joints, old injuries, over 60 or carrying extra weight, aqua exercise is a Godsend.

This isn't always what we see on TV. Weight loss is dramatized on shows where trainers demand very heavy people to take on intense workouts right away. I don't believe that this is healthy, or the right way to train. I've seen people on these shows who weigh 300 and 400 pounds forced to run on treadmills at six miles an hour. Some of these people fall off the treadmill, pass out and vomit. That's why there are always medics on hand.

Work out in a way that is challenging for where you're at. It's okay to start slow, and advance from there. In fact, this is the only way to go if you want to work out without injury for the rest of your life.

Start with a brisk walk outside, on the track or treadmill. Bring your earbuds, so that you can enjoy your tunes, and rock out. After a few weeks of the brisk walks, you can add a lap of jogging, or switch to a cardio machine that is more challenging. The point is to keep progressing because as you become more conditioned, you'll need new and interesting ways to move and stay in your cardio zone. You'll be addicted to how amazing movement and sweat feels; you won't be able to imagine your life without it. On the days you don't exercise, you'll miss it. What a beautiful addiction to replace the old days of no movement and garbage food!

"Take care of your body with steadfast fidelity. The soul must see through these eyes alone, and if they are dim, the whole world is clouded." -Goethe

Chapter 7

Essential Habits for Healthy Weight

What shape we're in depends on a few variables outside of diet and exercise. If you're not doing the right things in the areas of sleep, caffeine, stress reduction and who's on your support team, then improvements in diet and exercise will only go so far toward your healthy weight goals.

Get to sleep by 11:00 p.m.

The quantity and quality of sleep you get *effects your weight*. Looking at 18 studies done on how sleep effects weight and eating, researchers found that lack of sleep led to cravings for high-carb foods. Another study in the *American Journal of Clinical Nutrition* showed that people who were sleep deprived turned to late-night, high carb snacking.

I recommend getting into bed by 10:30 and falling asleep by 11:00 because the brain can most easily release sleep chemicals before that time. After 11:00, your brain has a much harder time releasing the chemicals that put you to sleep.

Get in bed by 10:00 or 10:30 with a book or lie with the lights out; no TVs, computers, phones or other sources of sounds and lights should be on, because these signal the brain that it's time to be alert.

Drift off to sleep by 11:00 p.m. latest. After a few nights of early-to-bed, you'll find that you rise in the morning feeling well-rested.

When you go to sleep by 11:00, you are set up for quality sleep cycles throughout the night. This ensures that the next day, you have the energy you need for home, work and exercise. When you are well-rested, you can think clearly, and get through the day with much more energy and joy.

Sleep-deprived people feel as though they're in a fog. They tell me that they're unable to make good decisions about what to eat, and how to fit exercise into their day. They've often gotten into the habit of going to bed late and only getting 4-5 hours of sleep.

There are a few things we can do in order to influence the ability to fall asleep: shut down our computers and phones at night, and stop drinking caffeine. Caffeine effects us for 12 hours after it's taken in, so if you want a good night's sleep, you'll have to stop drinking it by 11:00 a.m.

Stress reduction

To make the whole weight loss challenge even harder, how's this for a kick in the pants: your body can put on extra fat because of hormone levels in response to stress. This means that even while you change your diet and include exercise in your life, that *your own body can make itself fatter.*

If you have chronic stress, you may notice that the scale doesn't move in the right direction. This is maddening, but there is a simple, biological reason for it. A chronically stressed out person cannot lose weight because the body is trying to protect itself. Here's what happens:

First, the body releases cortisol when it is chronically stressed. The presence of cortisol in the bloodstream is a warning that the body is under duress. In response to this, the brain sends fatty cells to protect the body, because the brain cannot distinguish stress that is life threatening from stress that is not. The body takes the fatty cells and puts it around the mid-section, where the organs are, which we want to protect the most, then other places like the thighs and butt. This fat is not even coming from ice-cream or cake; it's coming from our own brains! The best way to provide comfort, the brain reasons, is by putting on layers of cushiony fat.

If you are experiencing chronic stress because of life events such as illness in the family, a negative work environment or a troubled relationship, know that these things are part of life for most people from time to time. The best we can do is to *provide relaxation and stress reduction for ourselves.*

Getting your exercise several times per week is essential for stress reduction, so be sure that you are getting in your cardio and strength workouts. The next step is to also take the time to do things that are relaxing for you personally. Even simple things like listening to your favorite CDs, reading, making a craft or getting together with a friend make a huge difference. Count on time to yourself to relax daily.

The people I know who practice regular meditation, tai chi or yoga are more centered, relaxed and happy, so I highly recommend finding such a practice if it's for you.

Next, add a massage or other spa treatment every couple of months. The therapeutic value of massage is amazing. My client, Mary Beth, gets a manicure every six weeks, and looks forward to it as a way of rewarding herself for sticking with 95 percent healthy eating and exercise.

There are many ways to reduce stress without using food. Find ways to let go of the stress and relax every day, and experience the great benefits. This self-care will make it possible to attain a healthy weight, so spend the time and money as an investment in yourself. You are worth it, and the people who love you will notice a big difference in your happiness, and in their relationships with you.

Don't go it alone

Look for at least one guide who can offer support and encouragement while you make these very important changes in your eating, exercise and weight. The world's best leaders have advisors and other accountability partners to help them stay motivated.

Because there are so many different coaches, nutritionists and trainers out there, find people who are qualified, helpful and invested in their clients. I encourage you to find at least one professional person to add to your team. Some good people to have on your team are: a friend who also has wellness goals, a caring and knowledgeable trainer at your gym, a life coach, a nutritionist or a class that focuses on both nutrition and exercise.

If you feel that having a nutritionist look at what you're eating and make recommendations would help, then find one who is going to emphasize real foods like lean meat and/or other protein sources, vegetables, fruits, nuts and seeds and one who educates people on reading food labels.

Reaching out for the support you need must come from the belief that you're worth it. You are! With the belief that your body, mind and spirit deserve nourishment, making the healthiest choice in any given moment becomes a way of life.

Remember that eating nourishing food, exercising and practicing stress reduction lead to healthy weight when practiced consistently. Make a list of the ideas in this book that resonated most with you, and do them daily. The little things add up and bring you to the big thing, which is healthy weight. *This is what I want for you*, so that you can live a life of inner peace and happiness, leaving fat prison, fatigue and body angst behind forever.

Please write to me and let me know how you're doing, at deniseroma@yahoo.com.

Acknowledgements

Thank you to the following people, who helped make this book a reality:

Book coach Kim O'Hara, for encouraging me, making me a better writer and showing me that this is not just another diet and exercise book, but a message that needs to be available to everyone out there struggling with the realities of body hate, diet failure and what it's like to be heavy and tired.

The fitness trainers and other extraordinary people in my McGaw YMCA family (Emily Rasmussen, Ryan Kish, Alyson Mann, Steve Seidel) for providing me the platform from which to learn what to eat, how to work out and finally break free from fat prison. I will always be grateful to these angels for being alongside me.

Editor Corrie Worou, who is brilliant.

Mary Lou Denardo, Cecelia Daspit, Judy Krizmanic, Amy Babinec and Jon Novi, for reading this book in various stages, and provided insights that influenced its development.

My mom, Shirley Roma, for showing me from the beginning that beauty is grace and kindness, even more so than healthy weight.

Jon Novi, for cooking us healthy dinners every single night, sending me off with a lunch and snacks every weekday and giving me more love than I thought I'd ever get.

All of the beautiful souls traveling this earth in bodies of various shapes and sizes, who I hope this book inspires to ditch the body hate, and start living…well in the 95 percent!